Prepare For Aging

The hard and stiff will be broken.

The soft and supple will prevail.

From Lao-Tzu, by Steven Mitchell

PREPARE

FOR

AGING

INSPIRATIONAL STORIES
TO KEEP YOU MOVING!

Dr. Kevin T Morgan

Senior Ironman Triathlete And Student Of Optimal
Movement

BookBaby Inc.

TRADEMARKS:

Any trademarks, service marks, product names or named features are assumed to be the property of their respective owners, and are used for reference only.

SHARING THIS DOCUMENT:

I politely ask that you please respect my work by not donating or reselling this book. This would be very much appreciated.

MEDICAL DISCLAIMER:

As a veterinarian, I do not provide medical advice to human animals. If you undertake or modify an exercise program, consult your medical advisers before doing so. Undertaking activities pursued by the author does not mean that he endorses your undertaking such activities, which is clearly your decision and responsibility. Be careful and sensible, please. Old Dogs in Training, LLC.

I dedicate this book by my good friend, and fellow triathlete,

Frits with an 's,' who left us recently.

Sorely missed!

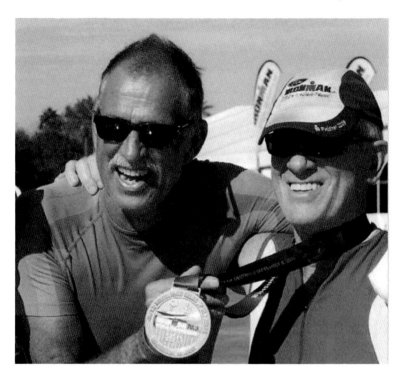

Frits, left, with the author, at the World Half Ironman Championships in Las Vegas, 2013. We lost a great triathlete and a wonderful person. Thanks for the "Ironman Training Secret Sauce," my friend. You continue to be an inspiration.

CONTENTS

PREPARE

FOR

AGING

INSPIRATIONAL STORIES
TO KEEP YOU MOVING!

AUTHOR'S NOTE

I suspect that the real trick to enjoying our 'Golden Years,' is to plan ahead. Such planning includes correction of life's chronic injuries, as best we can. Be they physical, intellectual, emotional, spiritual or interpersonal. The way to do this is to be open to changing and learning.

Adaptation to the physical challenges of aging is the subject of this book, which is presented in large part as the OQS Method. Observe, Question (the obvious), Solve, with or without professional guidance. This method grew out of my desire to complete a full Ironman race in my 50s. The sport of Ironman Triathlon became a way of life, much to my surprise. It still is, 20 years later - *go figure!*

Ironman is tough, aging is tougher!

As a scientific lecturer for many years, I learned that lectures don't work. Stories do! We are a story telling species, thus the use of stories in this book. Each story, from my life as a country vet and a research scientist, has been selected to provide a lesson.

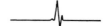

Each lesson made life easier, while enhancing my effectiveness and happiness. Many of these lessons are related to staying mobile and active, both mentally and physically.

My goal for you is that you enjoy your golden years to the full, which takes a little preparation.

Especially when comes to the way you move!

MIND-BODY OPTIMIZATION

The Observing, Questioning, Solving (OQS) Method.

Step One: *Observing*

You won't fix what you don't notice.

Step Two: *Questioning*

The pain may not be where the problem lies.

Step Three: *Solving*

First understand. Then solve.

Step Four: *Sitting*

Sit right to live right.

Step Five: *Standing*

Your body-movement laboratory.

Step Six: *Walking/Running*

You walk/run how you think and feel and *vice versa*!

NOTE:

If you want to jump straight into working on the way you move, read Appendix A: *On Balance*. Then go to

Appendix B: *Cliffs Notes Approach To Applying The OQS Method.*

Of course, I recommend that you read the entire narrative before doing so. It all depends how you like to do things.

We're all different; that's for sure!

INTERNET LINKS:

This book refers to a number of relevant Internet sites, including the author's YouTube channel. Sites that the author doesn't control can go down or change at anytime. All recommended links are indicated as (link), which you will find on the website dedicated to this book:

http://changethewayyoumove.info

This approach permits the author to refresh links that change or go down after publication.

PROLOGUE

If I had an hour to solve a problem, I'd spend 55 minutes thinking about the problem, and 5 minutes thinking about solutions. – Albert Einstein

Caring is the key! – FitOldDog

1970 on a cold winter's evening.

It's the end of a long day, tending to livestock. I'm ready for my dinner!

I'd been working as a country vet on farms in the Southwest of England for three years.

Tonight, an old farmer and I are in a cowshed by the light of a single, grimy light bulb. A bunch of old buildings, straw, hay, mud and hard work all around. Cobwebs hang from the rafters. Fifteen dairy cows, Jerseys, chewing the cud in the evening gloom. Delightful animals. Gentle as you can imagine and affectionate for cows.

This nice old guy is just getting by. That's for sure!

He's looking at me out of old, worried eyes, from a heavily wrinkled face. This man has seen, and is still living, hard times. But he cares about his livestock. I came to treat one of his cows for mastitis.

As I write the ticket for the bill, he says,

"I guess you can't do nowt for old Mabel, young man?"

I wasn't one of the owners of the veterinary practice. A hired hand, an assistant, as opposed to a partner in the business. I couldn't waste time or other resources.

"What's up with Mabel?" I replied. Which one was Mabel, I had no idea!

"She can't eat, and she's losing weight. Mabel's a family pet. She gave up giving milk years ago. We like to keep her around, you know!"

I took a look at Mabel. A kind soul. She had managed to break her mandibular symphysis. That's where the two halves of the lower jaw join together at the front. Fingers of bone on each side "interdigitate" to create a single solid structure. Imagine linking your hands by clasping your fingers. Left, right, left, right. That's how the mandibular symphysis works, combined with strong bands of dense connective tissue.

This nice old farmer doesn't have a lot of money. He doesn't want to send her off to slaughter either. She's a family friend. I racked my brains for an affordable – even free - solution. Major surgery, with plates and screws, would cost a lot, even if it was possible in an old dairy cow.

It was the end of a long day!

I'd earned my living and am about to head home. Then a thought strikes me! I can do this job, on my own time. A length of strong, absorbable suture material, cat gut (about 20 cents). Local anesthetic (another 20 cents), and a drug to keep her calm (50 cents). I'd see if I could pull that jaw back together. It'll be a tough job, but I'll give it a go!

I'll clean out the joint and bind the two halves together with a figure-of-eight suture knot. Imagine someone passing string around the palms of your hands in a figure of eight. Over the top of the right hand. Down and under your left. Then over the top of your left, then down and under your right. Several turns to pull your hands, and thus your opposing fingers, together. The only difference is the rigid nature of jaw bones and the unpredictable behavior of a cow's head!

Could I pass the cat gut under the jaw bones without damaging any nerves or crushing blood vessels? Back to my memories of cow anatomy - should be fine. That's what we did, that kind, old farmer and I. He distracted Mabel. I performed the surgery, crude as it was.

Only took about an hour!

I came back two weeks later. The farmer was delighted, welcoming me with open arms, in a subdued,

Somerset-Farmer way. Mabel was happy, putting on weight again. The case of mastitis had cleared up too. That old cow was saved for a buck or so, with a little thought and some surgical experience, by:

Observing *the problem* - What did this observation process involve? Well! The cow's jaw, for sure. Then the general state of the cow. Could Mabel handle the intended surgery. Then there was the farmer, his financial situation and concern for Mabel, as an old friend. There was also my relationship to the farmer and the veterinary practice, which led me to do this work inexpensively on my own time. There was also my level of surgical experience. Could I take on such a surgery. Clearly, observation needs to include the entire context of the situation, as it will for you as you tackle the challenges of aging.

Questioning *potential surgical approaches* - This was a simpler issue, as the choices were limited to do nothing, send her to the experts at the local veterinary school, or work it out for myself. It will be the same for you with the physical strains of exercise as you age: hope the pain goes away, consult a medical expert, or work out how to fix the issue yourself. The answer can be simple or not so simple, as you will see in this book.

Solving *Mabel's dilemma* - This is always the goal, to solve the problem, whether it's fixing a struggling cow or repairing a calf strain.

*And finally, **helping** that old farmer, affordably.*

Why do I consider affordability to be important, when it comes to adapting to aging? Because we don't all have health insurance, and even if we do the co-pays can drain our bank account. Cost should be factored into the process of adapting to aging, but not to the point of risking one's life. This takes a little thought, patience and experience, that's all.

These are the basics of the method presented in this book . . . *to help you to change the way you think and move, while considering all of the relevant variables.*

I know I sound like a scientist, I can't help it. I just love science!

GOLDEN YEARS?

It is not the strongest of the species that survives, nor the most intelligent. It is the one that is most adaptable to change. – Charles Darwin

Golden Years?

You must be joking! Who do you think came up with this expression?

"The term "Golden Years" was coined in 1959, as an advertising pitch for Sun City, " Robert R. Rowley, PS says. It worked for their business!

But for us? Give us a break!

The 'golden years' are tough! Money is tighter, for most. Young people don't listen to us anymore. Aches and pains, where you never had aches and pains in the morning on getting out of bed. Why am I so stiff? Furthermore, technology changes so fast that it's hard to keep up.

Then diabetes or heart disease. Your friends start to die. (I lost two friends recently)

Then my cancer surgery two months ago. Today my left hip flexor (iliacus) is so tight I can't run, and I can't read a damned thing without my glasses.

But I'm happy! Why is that?

Happiness is a choice for most of us! There's always 'good' and 'bad' stuff going on, so I try to focus on the good stuff.

I use brief meditations - as in The Five Minute Meditator by David Harp - throughout the day. This allows me to stay in the moment, or as Eckhart Tolle would put it, The Now! This practice has a calming effect. It relaxes my body and improves the fluidity of my movements.

I have things to wake up for in the morning! I do things! I love life! I'm lucky that way!

I also adapt as best I can to 'aging decay' to continue the adventure! Aging and death are inevitable. That doesn't mean we need to hurry them along!

You may have to change the way you think and move!

INTRODUCTION

My Beloved Sport Saved by the
Study of Optimal
Body Movement

In the beginner's mind, there are many possibilities. In the expert's mind, there are few.

– Shunryu Suzuki

September 2010.

I'm sitting alone in a hotel room in Barcelona, Spain. Here to visit my Mom, who continued to be active and healthy into her 90s.

I'm wondering what to do!

I'd completed my fourth Lake Placid Ironman (2.4-mile swim, 112-mile bike ride, 26.2-mile run) in June, only a few months previously. My best race time yet: 13 hours and 34 minutes. I even came in, in the daylight. A first!

That race saved my life!

On race day I was 67 years old and as fit as I'd ever been. Trained by a great coach, Chris Hauth. First out of the water in my age group (65-69). I head off on the bike, feeling strong as an ox. At mile 30, I hear a voice, "Hey! You're in my age group [it's written on my calf!]. How's it going? My name's Frits. Frits with an s." We chat and later become good friends.

Frits is a powerful cyclist. He heads off into the distance, but Ironman, like aging, is unforgiving; you have to pace yourself! I think, *He's a big guy. He's going to crash and burn on the run. He's going too fast!* That's exactly what happened. Frits informs me three years later, when we meet at another race in Las Vegas.

I'm off the bike, 40 minutes ahead of my only real competition. Everything is going according to plan but then the big surprise. Horrendous foot pain at about 10 miles into the run. A burning sensation on the soles of both feet. I've never experienced this before. If I walk, it goes away. If I try to run, back it comes almost immediately. I'm forced to slow down, to hobble along. At mile 137 a great runner, Roger, slips by me. I remember thinking, *I wish I could run like that.* He'd pulled up the 40 minutes and went on to gain another 12 on me before the 140.2-mile finish line.

There goes my Kona slot!

The reward for finishing first in your age group is a place in the Ironman World Championships in Hawaii. I was expecting a 4-hour, 15-minute marathon, but I took over 5 hours with my foot pain. I couldn't run, in spite of friends egging me on, as I came within a couple of miles of the finish line!

That foot pain saved my life!

After returning home from the race, I was lying in bed wondering, *What the h*ll happened. It was in the bag!*

Being a pathologist by training, I review my symptoms (**Observing!**). A mild abdominal pulse which I'd noticed and discounted the previous January. At that time my resting pulse was 38 beats per minute. I had a huge stroke volume, the amount of blood pumped out of the heart on each beat. This creates a prominent pulse, which is easier to feel in lean race-shape. I assumed my 'abdominal pulse' was due to a blood vessel in my gut. Then there was that weird foot pain in the race (**Questioning**). On the soles of my feet as far away from my heart as you can get, thus, furthest from the source of drive pressure.

Cancer? The most likely choice at my age, 67. I'm using logic, as feelings generally have no place in the diagnostic process.

Not cancer! Nothing fits.

Next on my diagnostic list? An abdominal aortic aneurysm (AAA). The squishy pulse, loss of 'feed pressure' for blood to my feet. I look down at my belly. It's moving up and down with each heart beat. It all makes sense. An AAA! A big one. About to blow!

If it ruptures, I'll be dead in minutes.

An ultrasound exam, the next day, reveals my diagnosis to be correct. A 6.9 cm. diameter bulge in my aorta. I have no idea how it survived that race. Especially those climbs on the bike during the last 15 miles as you approach the end of the bike course. Baby Bear, Momma Bear and Daddy Bear, each tougher than the last!

A few days later, I'm undergoing surgery for the insertion of an AAA stent graft (**Solving!**). This is a large plastic and metal tube about seven inches long. It's an inch wide at the top with spikes, just like grappling hooks, to hold it in place near my kidneys. At the bottom, there are two smaller branches that supply blood to my legs. (Go to Zenith Flex AAA Endovascular Graft on YouTube, to watch how it's done.) This remarkable piece of engineering was inserted into my aorta via an artery in my leg. The aorta is the biggest artery in your body. It connects the heart to your organs, muscles, and everything else.

From now on, I have to trust my life to this internal crutch, the AAA stent graft. I named my stent Rupert, after Rupert Bear, a childhood story character. Why not? We're a team now.

For a few days after the surgery, I was pretty depressed. That's normal.

It's a big change. I'm only human!

In my mind I'd gone from Ironman-Distance Triathlete Scientist to aortic cripple!

Within a few weeks, I recover from surgery and am feeling pretty normal again. The problem with aortic aneurysms is that you can't feel them until they are about to rupture. I can't feel Rupert, either – I'm glad. It might creep me out!

Can I continue my beloved Ironman training with an AAA stent graft?

I ask the surgeon, Joe, what he thinks. I can tell that he had serious reservations. All Joe said was, "Well, I'd go easy, at first, if it was me!" It was clear that Joe wouldn't go there if it was him. Joe did complete an Ironman, a couple of years later. Not with an AAA stent graft, fortunately. He told me he'd never put himself through that again - this is a common response! Usually half the field, of up to 3,000 athletes, will only finish one full Ironman race.

I love the Ironman lifestyle, generally doing one per year. People ask me why I do it. My response is always the same, "It keeps me out of assisted living!"

I continued to seek the input of doctors and surgeons, in person and online. Each one indicated verbally, with a frown, or with silence, that it would be ill-advised. I received no further advice or guidance. I was on my own! Since then I've heard the same refrain from other athletes with vascular disease (link).

I wondered: *Are these medical experts right? Should I give up my beloved sport? Do they know? Or should I risk my life, for my Ironman training lifestyle? What's to do?*

Then I remembered one of my favorite mantras:

A life without risk is no life at all!

With a little trepidation, I decided to set aside the conservative recommendations of doctors and surgeons. To consider going ahead with my training for the Lake Placid Ironman 2011. The medical profession can only provide limited guidance to people, such as myself. It really is up to each of us to work out how to live our lives! Maybe I can make some changes in my training to protect my stent graft. For instance, I wonder if there are reports of AAA stent graft displacement or damage due to mechanical stresses that may provide me with some guidance and insights.

[In 2013, I demonstrated that an AAA stent graft can be dislocated in a bike wreck, but that's another story]

In that hotel room, I had to grapple with how to safely continue Ironman training, with an AAA stent graft? This is a classic benefit-risk problem! The benefits need to outweigh the risks, or it's not worth it! My thoughts went like this, *To keep myself safe, and reduce the risk of displacing Rupert, I have to find a solution! To find a solution, I have to fully understand the problem. Thank goodness I have medical training, a definite advantage. I've seen aortas of all shapes and sizes as a veterinary pathologist. It can't be that difficult!*

Years later, I converted these thoughts and my subsequent experiences into a simple equation. It can be found on my blog under the title, *Sport Benefit Risk Analysis: Rediscovering Your Sport Safely After A Major Health Challenge* (link).

Of course, I don't know what I'm in for as I sit alone in my hotel room in Barcelona. Will I kill myself as I attempt to return to my sport? What I needed was a mentor, but none existed, at least none that I could find. Later, I would go on to guide others, with aortic or heart disease, on the return to their favorite physical activity or sport.

I'll see what I can find on the Internet.

Nothing!

Then, I wondered, *What if I start a blog? Other Ironman-distance triathletes with AAA stent grafts will get in touch.*

I write my first blog post after struggling to master hosting and set up my site, Athlete With Stent. It feels like throwing a bottle with a message into the sea. First, I blog about training with an AAA stent graft. Then, I write about Ironman experiences as an older athlete. Finally, I write about philosophy and the meaning of life. But no other

Ironman-distance triathlete with an AAA stent graft ever does turn up. Victor, my 'bike guy,' says to me one day, "Kevin, they may all be dead. I think you dodged a bullet!"

I knew the benefits of Ironman racing: the pleasure of training, racing with my son, being alive.

But what about the risks?

I studied the structure of my stent! I found an article that reported AAA stent graft dislocation. With severe injury or death in several instances. One due to intense rowing. Another following a Heimlich Maneuver, and several due to car lap belts during a wreck. You can imagine how confident that made me feel. I wish this information had been part of my discharge forms upon leaving the hospital.

There was nothing out there about athletes with AAA stents. There didn't seem to be a system for it. We are a rare breed, athletes with AAA stents.

On returning home from Spain, I made my decision.

It's time to train for the 2011 Lake Placid Ironman.

I consulted with engineers involved in the construction of AAA stent grafts. I investigated the risk of metal fatigue and other factors that might dislocate or damage it and kill me. This research led to calculated modifications to my usual Ironman training plan.

I had to change the way I moved!

Reduce hip flexion: To avoid pulling on the arteries containing the stent graft.

- An elliptical trainer replaced the rowing machine for warm-ups in the gym. That was a loss, as I enjoyed the rowing machine!

- A bike, designed to reduce hip flexion, was constructed by Victor Jimenez of BicycleLab. She fits like a glove!

- Quit flip turns in the pool. No loss. How many flip turns do you do in an open water swim? Zero!

- Shorter pedal cranks? They weren't available for Victors' bike design!

Minimize impact stresses: To reduce the risk of stent displacement.

- Low impact running, which I'd already mastered for other reasons.

- Standing off the saddle on the bike on bumpy roads.

Focus on volume, rather than intensity: Avoid excessive expansion and contraction of my aorta.

- More long steady workouts.

- Avoid excessive loads.

It's basically endurance training. This is better for older athletes with or without vascular disease.

If you want to keep an old car (guy) running, drive it (him) gently!

One year later, in 2011, Rupert and I completed the Lake Placid Ironman. Three hours slower than in 2010 but feeling great. We appear to be the only ones to do so, so far at least (link). This is not a claim to fame I recommend!

How was this victory achieved, apart from the work of all the people who invented, built and inserted that AAA stent graft? It was done by,

Observing the way my body moves, in the swim, the bike and the run.

Questioning the decision as a benefit/risk issue.

Solving the problem by modifying movement.

Adapting to the new circumstances.

I simply changed the way I moved!

SIX SIMPLE STEPS

The six steps are based on my journey and the insights of people who have shared their personal stories. You will encounter both mental and physical roadblocks, as you adapt to aging.

This book was designed to help you succeed.

Not everyone has the money for private Yoga or Feldenkrais lessons or even classes. Many don't have health insurance, but they still want to enjoy an active lifestyle. Most of us, like myself, are generally unaware of how we move, even later in life. Being well-paid at the time, I invested thousands of dollars and hundreds of hours into body movement training. From martial arts to Yoga. Aging changes that! Money is an issue later in life. Unless you are fortunate enough to become independent of a paycheck.

Unnecessary trips to a doctor or physical therapist can break the bank. Since retiring from my career as a scientist, I miss those paychecks. Now I'm working to build a business, to help people with the challenges of aging. There is no guarantee of success in business, so money is an issue.

That said, if I need help, I seek it. For instance, a few years ago, I suffered a spasm of the *gluteus minimus,* a small hip muscle. It was throwing my pelvis out of line. I couldn't get it to let go with all that body movement training. An excellent physical therapist applied dry needling - unpleasant, but it worked. That pesky muscle let go, finally. The problem is knowing when to seek help and when to fix it on your own.

Only you can decide, but if you know your body you'll have a better chance of getting it right!

The entrepreneur's life, like aging, is not for the faint of heart. But it gets me out of bed and ready to rock and roll, every morning. Such challenges are typical for most of us, in our so-called golden years. That said, I'm finding that they are golden. The gold is in being able to help other people. From time to time I receive thanks for my work. Having changed someone's life for the better. Here is what 'Jim The Runner' had to say, about my first book, *Surgery Recovery Guide, Based On My Abdominal Aortic Aneurysm Experience:*

"After you read this book, it will give you confidence that you too can get your life back. It worked for me. I am back running again and I love it."

This made me feel great, and the $6.94 royalty check helped too!

You don't have to give into the idea that aging will prevent you from having adventures. They may not include climbing Everest. But they might! For some, a long day-hike is plenty and very rewarding. For others, getting to the restroom unaided is a challenge. You feel like you deserve a medal. We each have to find our element when it comes to our chosen activities, including sports. If you don't enjoy what you do, you won't stick at it. It's a fact of life. For some people, that's the hardest part of exercise, finding enjoyment in it!

The first three chapters of this book explain the Observing, Questioning, Solving (OQS) Method. The next three chapters apply these skills to our three major activities: sitting, standing and walking/running.

Step One: **Observing** - Observation, like listening, is a valuable skill. We are surrounded by distractions. Watch those people running trails in the woods on a beautiful day. Flowers, birds, signs of wildlife all around. They're zoned out, listening to music, or worse still a podcast. Say "Hi! Lovely day!" and they don't hear you. They aren't actually in the woods, in nature, nor are they in their bodies. This is when injuries occur due to distraction and failure to focus on the job in hand. People have been killed, while running the roads distracted by ear buds.

Observational skills, leading to awareness, are critical for your future. Especially if you want to change the way you move, in a constructive, life-enhancing manner. Try to be like Sherlock Holmes and see what others miss.

Step Two: **Questioning** - Don't blindly follow your underlying assumptions. The problem may not be where the pain is. Finding the primary cause(s) of exercise stresses can involve detective work. If you can't work out what is going on, a good place to start is to change the way you move and see what happens. Remember, you're the detective!

Step Three: **Solving** - Facing change requires dealing with the new and different. The clearest example is how much longer it takes to recover from stresses and strains as you age.

The only way to get it right, with or without professional guidance, is to listen to your body. It's sending you messages all the time! Listen, learn and find solutions, by working to understand the problem **before** you try to fix it!

I call this the Observing, Questioning, Solving, or OQS, Method.

You then learn, in chapters four, five and six, how to apply OQS to your most common activities.

Step Four: **Sitting**

Step Five: **Standing**

Step Six: **Walking/Running**

We do these all the time and hope to do so far into our 'golden years.'

Yes! Sitting and standing are movement activities. How you undertake them will determine, at least in part, your state of health. Both mental and physical! For instance, standing in line becomes an opportunity to learn more about how you move, rather than a burden.

In the remaining pages of this book, we'll explore the process of realigning your body to overcome old habits. To repair damage we've done unconsciously, over the years. We'll consider the use of gravity and spinal elasticity for efficient movement. This will take you into the world of beginner's mind, where you can reinvent yourself. You will start collecting stories to tell your children, grandchildren and friends. Isn't that, to some degree, what life is about? We are a story-telling species.

Instructional tales have been used as analogies throughout this book. They come from my life as a country veterinarian in the 1970s, and as a scientist for the subsequent 40 years. As an English country vet, my life was much like those tales of James Herriot in *All Creatures Great And Small*. On the small farms of England. Back then the cows had names, not numbers. This is why I chose the beloved cow, Mabel, as an introduction to the OQS Method. You have to care about your body, in the same way that old farmer cared about Mabel.

My goal for you?

To bring your body movements into the light of consciousness, affordably!

Why affordably?

I want this to be open to anyone prepared to put in the effort. Rich or poor, of any educational level and physical ability. When it comes to the six steps, it will cost you as much as you wish to invest. For OQS? Minimally $2-5, plus whatever you paid for this book.

That said, let's begin your mind-body movement journey!

PART ONE: THE THREE OQS TOOLS

Observing, Questioning, Solving

CHAPTER ONE

THE FIRST STEP

OBSERVING

To acquire knowledge, one must study; but to acquire wisdom, one must observe.

– Marilyn Vos Savant

It's the fall of 1963.

I hear someone screaming.

I'm confused, but I wonder if they need help. I'm lying on the ground. Dazed! Then I realize there are two screams. One is from my full-throttle motorbike engine. The other is from me! I stop screaming and pass out!

I've been hit by a car.

I'm in Bristol, England. A teenager. An experienced motorcyclist. I had traveled over 200 miles the previous day. On busy highways, from Lincolnshire in the North of England to Bristol in the Southwest. In pouring rain. Slick busy roads. Now, on a sunny, Saturday morning, I'm making a five-minute trip to a friend's house on my BSA Gold Flash, 650-Twin motorbike. What a bike! Light traffic on a regular street in my old neighborhood. Nineteen years old, a cautious rider, aware of his surroundings.

Nothing can go wrong!

Something catches my attention. I glance to my right. A large car is headed straight for me from a side road. The driver is not looking my way. In fact, he's facing towards the back seat. It turns out that he was trying to stop his kids from fighting. I can relate to this now, having had three of my own! The car slams into my side. I fly through the air, making a complete somersault, before hitting the road. A somersault was no new thing to me, but my competition diving career is terminated in an instant. I bounce along the road and roll up onto the sidewalk. Fortunately, I pass out from the pain and shock.

More than 40 years later, I learn a lot from this accident. About body-awareness and how to keep my much older body moving.

Physical accidents leave an archeological record in your body. One's immediate reaction is to protect or guard the injury. We tense our muscles to immobilize the affected area, to prevent further damage and pain. The problem with this short-term strategy? It can become long-term. Locked into our behavior patterns, as guarding, or chronic psychosomatic tension. Such tension can induce body movement problems later in life. In my case, much later in life! Thus, my enthusiasm for body awareness and optimal movement training.

As a scientist, I embraced a wide range of scientific disciplines.

Scientific disciplines are tools. We create them to make scientific discovery possible. Human brains are limited. The Universe is infinite in its complexity. The field of chemistry is no more real to the Universe than the country known as England. They are both products of human imagination. Doomed to be enlightening (or not) figments of the human experience.

Why is this important for your health?

Because medical science disciplines are fragmented. The average family doctor knows little about the mechanics of body movement. Compared to a sports physician, osteopathic doctor or physical therapist. If you have a problem with your feet, do you go to a podiatrist? A chiropractor? Yoga instructor, sports physician, physical therapist, or your local shoe store? How do you decide? They will all say, "Come to me!" I've been to most of them in my body movement journey.

How to choose where to go? Of whom to ask advice? This is challenging, especially with limited financial resources.

This book will help you to unscramble this puzzle, to some extent. It will still involve some trial, error and guess work on your part.

Rule #1

Suspend your trust in the obvious - a whole new way of thinking!

It's easy to assume that pain is where the problem lies. For instance, pain in your left arm may indicate trouble with your heart. The same applies to many muscle and joint pains. I encountered this assumption with a severe case of running-induced knee pain in my 60s.

As a youngster I was a swimmer, not a runner.

What you do as a kid can affect what you can do as an adult. We store the body memory, from childhood and teenage athletics, into adulthood. Ride a bike or swim, as a youngster, and those skills remain available as body memories. Throughout your life! Such abilities are more challenging to create from scratch, as an adult.

It's the same with languages. Learned as a child, perfect! Learned as an adult, you almost always have a foreign accent and make minor mistakes of gender and the like. This I know, from my studies of French as an adult in Geneva, Switzerland. Our young kids embraced the language in a way I never could. In months they had no accent or gender errors. Compared to my years of persistent study, but imperfect skills.

What has this to do with my teenage motorbike wreck and body movement?

A great deal!

Let's go to the summer of 2001.

I'm in my late 50s. I decided I wanted to complete an Ironman race. I was watching my youngest son in the Lake Placid Ironman. Mesmerized by the energy of the start. Three thousand athletes, of all ages, lined up in Mirror Lake, awaiting the gun at 7:00 am. Um! Sitting in a cold lake at 7:00 a.m. is not my favorite part. But the energy of the competitors and the excitement of the crowd sucked me in. I watched my son go by on the bike and the run. About 10 hours later he made the final turn at the High School Stadium. To a cheering crowd and YOU ARE AN IRONMAN! from the loud speakers.

I thought, *I'd like to do that!*

Little did I know what I was letting myself in for! A full Ironman race includes a 2.4-mile swim, 112-mile bike ride, and a 26.2-mile marathon, all in one day. If there were any weak links in my physical and mental chains, that would reveal them. Reveal them it did.

First step! Tackling long distance swimming. As a water polo player for 10 years as a youngster, I was well trained for sprinting. Not for long-haul, open-water swimming. I found the Total Immersion Swimming Technique on the web (link). It's great for improving your balance in the water. With a little work my long-distance swims were up to snuff.

Then I bought a triathlon bike and started riding longer and longer distances. I cycled a lot as a youngster. This was tough training, but doable.

But I'd never been a runner.

I didn't enjoy running. I didn't seem to have the stamina for it, especially in my legs. Having had mild rickets as a toddler, due to a vitamin deficiency. One of the effects of World War II. Born in 1943, 18 months before the end of the war. Even though Mum did a great job, food, especially good food, was scarce for the first 10 years of my life. War is hard on kids, nutritionally and in many other ways.

You can't complete an Ironman without learning how to run a marathon on tired legs. I took lessons from my triathlete son. He said I ran like a loaf of bread. Correct! I had no idea how to run or engage my whole body in the process. I hired a triathlete coach and took running lessons, gradually increasing the distance. On reaching 5 miles, my right knee would express extreme distress. Knee pain! The deep, throbbing, "you have to stop running" kind!

I had to fix it to complete the 26.2-mile run segment of my Ironman dream.

Over the next year, I tried everything I could think of to cure that running-induced knee pain. Including the gold standard of rest, ice and stretching. By the way, when you're stretching think lengthening. This isn't something you do TO your body; it's a conversation WITH your body. Furthermore, don't focus on a muscle; place your attention on the action. To lengthen your hamstrings, focus on the act of reaching towards your toes. Never force it! 'Stretching' is an art (link)!

Unable to fix it on my own, I sought professional medical assistance:

- Two chiropractors ($450)

- A sports massage therapist ($600)

- A yoga instructor ($300)

- A kinesiologist ($80)

- An acupuncturist ($120)

- Several podiatrists who sold me some expensive orthotics ($800)

- Two physical therapists ($650)

- Several doctors ($120 - copays)

- Finally, a sports medicine physician injected cortisone into my knee ($20 copay)

Thousands of dollars and nothing to show for it! I still couldn't run more than five miles pain-free.

Were my Ironman dreams over?

Then, by chance, I ran into Karen Dold. We knew each other from the world of science. Karen informed me that she'd abandoned Molecular Biology to teach the Feldenkrais Method. I literally said, without thinking, "What? The Frankenstein Method?" When it comes to marketing, this remarkable technique suffers from a terrible name.

Karen explained that Moshe Feldenkrais suffered a serious knee injury while playing soccer. He studied his problem, and created a new method of movement therapy. Moshe also succeeded in returning to his beloved soccer. The Feldenkrais Method is widely used today for recovery from many different sports injuries and physical challenges. Professional athletes and musicians use Feldenkrais to improve their performance.

I said, "Can you fix my knee?" Explaining my dilemma.

The following week I arrived at Karen's house, expecting another failure for my $70. First, Karen asked me to walk around her home office, while she watched every move I made. Then she said, "Stand in front of me, relax and sway from side to side." I did as instructed.

Then!

My understanding of body movement changed forever. "Kevin, do you know that when you sway to the left your body remains straight? When you sway to the right, your shoulders rotate a little. To bring your right shoulder forward a few millimeters."

I looked down and there it was! *But what does it mean!* I wondered?

Karen asked, "Have you had any serious accidents in the past?"

"Well, I did have a motorcycle wreck, about 40 years ago, which broke my right ankle."

"I suspect that you're guarding, or locking up, your right ankle. This forces your body to turn around your hips as you sway to the right. Do you have more trouble balancing on your right leg?"

The jig was up!

I'd been guarding that right ankle ever since that motorbike wreck. Completely unawares! It had no effect on walking or cycling, but running is less forgiving as is balancing on one leg. My knee pain was due to an issue with my ankle, believe it or not! Everyone else, including myself and all the medical professionals I consulted, assumed the problem was in my knee! Except my Feldenkrais Instructor.

Karen carefully **observed** the way I moved, with no such assumption!

Two millimeter rotation of my shoulders, less than the thickness of a couple of quarters. This tiny movement revealed the source of my knee problem. It directed me towards my ankle, my accident history, and the study of body awareness.

*It was time to **question** the way I moved!*

CHAPTER TWO

THE SECOND STEP

QUESTIONING

It ain't what you don't know that gets you into trouble. It's what you know for sure that just ain't so.

– Mark Twain

The year, 1846.

A salutary tale of a powerful observation, ignored. *Extracted from an article, by Rebecca Davis of North Carolina Public Radio.*

"Our hero is Ignaz Semmelweis, a Hungarian doctor. He wondered why so many women in maternity wards were dying from puerperal fever, also known as childbed fever. He studied two maternity wards in the hospital. One staffed by male doctors and medical students and the other by female midwives. He counted the number of deaths on each ward.

He noticed that more women were dying in the doctors' clinic than in the midwives' clinic. He tested things that may have been responsible. Whether the women delivered on their back or their side. Whether a priest passed through the ward, ringing a bell. Finally, Semmelweis hypothesized that there were cadaverous particles. Little pieces of corpse. That doctors and students were getting on their hands from the bodies they dissected. During delivery, these particles would get inside the women. Causing the women to develop the disease and die.

[NOTE: The germ theory of disease developed many years later].

If Semmelweis' idea was correct, getting rid of those particles should cut down on the death rate.

He ordered medical staff to start cleaning their hands and instruments. With a chlorine solution. Chlorine, as we know today, is about the best disinfectant there is. He chose chlorine because he thought it would be the best way to get rid of any smell.

The rate of childbed fever fell dramatically.

You'd think everyone would be thrilled. Semmelweis had solved the problem! But they weren't thrilled. Did he think the doctors were responsible for transmitting childbed fever to their patients? And Semmelweis wasn't tactful. He berated people who disagreed with him and made some influential enemies. The doctors gave up the chlorine hand-washing, and Semmelweis lost his job."

Those physicians knew they could not be transmitting diseases to their patients. It was obvious! They were doctors for heaven's sake. Get rid of that guy!

The Summer of 2016.

I'm reminded of Ignaz Semmelweis. I had recently published a report, based on several years research. On the underlying cause of so-called plantar fasciitis, aka acute morning heel pain. The report is available for download at Freedom From Foot Pain (link). It was a long, fascinating and frustrating journey. Like Semmelweis, I went from one idea to another. First, tight calf muscles. Next, an issue with connective tissue (fascia). I finally concluded that this condition originates in the nervous system. As a nociceptive response.

Nociception is the sensory nervous system's response to certain harmful stimuli.

I received insults for my trouble! Isn't that interesting? When you touch a nerve, you know there's a nerve to touch!

A fellow scientist said my work was junk science. A podiatrist wrote on social media that this research was based on BS. I wasn't fazed. That's science! Been there! Done that!

My mind drifts back to a winter's day in 1974.

I'm in a sparse government research office in Edinburgh, Scotland. Awaiting a visitor. The famous Dr. M. An established researcher and author in the field of brain diseases of farm animals. I had just published my first scientific article, "An Ultrastructural Study of Ovine Polioencephalomalacia" in the *Journal of Pathology*. The article cited his publications, favorably. I admired the man's work but had never met him. A formal letter arrived, stating that he would like visit and discuss the conclusions I had drawn in this publication.

Dr. M. was going to visit me! A beginner with only a few years' experience in brain research. I was looking forward to meeting the great man. To discussing our work. Especially brain biochemistry. I anticipated the debate with relish; it's how you learn!

Dr. M. knocks on my door and enters without ado. A dour powerful-looking man. Hanging up his dripping-wet raincoat, he rejects my offer of a hot cup of tea. He sits and observes me without expression. Clearly, things were not as expected. I ask after his 200-mile train journey and subsequent 5-mile bus trip. Silence!

His first words are,

"Why, exactly, do you presume to declare that the primary biochemical lesion of cerebro-cortical necrosis lies within the astrocyte?"

Well, at least he's read my paper.

He's pissed. Dr. M. had delivered a well-rehearsed three-pronged attack.

"Why, exactly, do you presume. . ." He was Dr. M. and I was just Mr. Morgan. My doctoral defense was one year hence. He was addressing a lower mortal.

"Cerebro-Cortical Necrosis" is the English name for this sheep disease. As opposed to the American term, Polioencephalomalacia - a more accurate description. I successfully defended this point of view at my PhD defense one year later.

"Lies within the astrocyte?" Dr. M. had postulated a primary neuronal (nerve cell) mechanism for this disease, with which my research results and logic conflicted. Who was I to disagree with the great Dr. M.?

We failed to resolve our differences. Dr. M. missed an opportunity to guide a young researcher. It's not a competition! This led me to write out a quote from *Zen And The Art Of Motorcycle Maintenance, An Inquiry Into Values*, by Robert M. Pirsig: "Any effort that has self-glorification as its final endpoint is bound to end in disaster." I taped it over my desk, where it remained for many years. Lest I forget this valuable lesson

Don't attack the person! Challenge their ideas, if it is appropriate to do so. Both logic and emotion are valuable tools in such a debate. Be sure you have a deep understanding of the subject matter or remain silent!

It doesn't matter who's right. It only what's right!

This is how I approached my research on so-called plantar fasciitis. I was surprised to find myself challenging ideas promoted by highly respected sources of medical advice. Including the Mayo Clinic and John Hopkins University. Disagreeing openly, with experts. Including the podiatrist who said my work was based on BS. My logic circuits love this kind of conflict. It never feels personal, just interesting!

Isn't it by questioning that medical science advances?

However! When it comes to our health care in the 'Western World', advertising budgets often play a bigger role than research budgets.

Can you guess how I finally fixed my morning heel pain?

By **observing**, **questioning** (the obvious), and **solving**. *By changing the way I moved,* as you will see.

Acute morning heel pain?

The experts will say you probably have plantar fasciitis. There are many, generally expensive, treatments for so-called plantar fasciitis, advertised on the Internet. One treatment, preferred by many doctors, is to inject cortisone into your heel. This is a bad idea! Why? Injections have the potential to cause infection. Furthermore, research has shown that any benefits last no more than four weeks.

I now understand how Ignaz must have felt!

My goal is to encourage you to learn how to read your body. To recognize subtle movements and behaviors. To discover how changing the way you move may provide benefit. To distinguish an open-minded physician from one stuck in a false paradigm.

My five years of heel-pain research in a nutshell:

2011: I awoke one morning, put my feet on the floor, and thought I had a shard of glass in my heel. I had acute, morning heel pain. I cured it by using a roller on my calf combined with hamstring stretches and single leg calf raises. So was the pain due to tight calves?

2012: I became suspicious of the term *plantar fasciitis*. The initial, acute pain is in the heel, not along the sole of the foot, in the region of the plantar fascia. I concluded that it is a progressive condition that first arises as intense heel pain. It involves the plantar fascia only in the latest stages of its progression, if at all.

2014: I had my second attack of heel pain. I cured it with the help of an Osteopathic Doctor. He realigned my displaced pelvis, which I'd suffered in a bicycle wreck in 2013. I then applied stretching, rolling, massage, and a movement modification. This modification I learned while testing the ASTRO (link). The design of this mechanical device is wisely based on studies of body movement.

I later made a simple observation about my heel pain. It was an observation made on myself. An anecdote to many. This observation was not the product of a large double-blind study. Supported by generous research funding. Was it science? Or was it junk science based on BS, I wondered? Then I remembered the story of John Snow and the pump handle.

In 1854, Dr. John Snow suspected that water from a public pump was the cause of a deadly cholera outbreak. He asked the district elders to have the pump handle removed, based on this hunch. After much debate, they followed Dr. Snow's advice. This contrasted starkly with the case of poor old Ignaz Semmelweis and childbed fever. The cholera outbreak ceased! This single action led to the realization that cholera spreads in drinking water. Was this an anecdote? Junk science based on a BS hunch? Or simply research!

Anyone can do research. Some of the best researchers I encountered didn't have PhD after their name. They possessed something much more valuable. Curiosity.

The problem comes when attempting to change people's minds. Whether you are right or wrong. They call it marketing! This book is a form of marketing. It's designed, at least in part, to replace drugs when appropriate, with lifestyle changes.

An Acute Morning Heel Pain Epiphany.

Though not as prestigious a person as the Drs. Ignaz Semmelweis or John Snow, I had an epiphany of my own. My second attack of morning heel pain was a rare opportunity to do some research. Pelvis realigned and symptoms beginning to resolve. It was time to question the true nature of this condition.

An epiphany: I soon observed that I could induce the characteristic stabbing heel pain by sitting on my hamstrings for a few minutes! At anytime during the day. I then discovered that I could quickly end this discomfort by stretching the hamstring muscles of the affected leg. Such an observation is inconsistent with the prevailing view that this condition is due to inflammation of the plantar fascia.

As scientists are wont to do, I came up with a hypothesis, as follows:

So-called plantar fasciitis is a progressive condition. In its early stages, it is a nociceptive, or neural (nervous system), response to body movement stresses. A warning of worse to come, including tissue damage, if you don't change the way you move!

Acute morning heel pain is best treated by *changing the way one moves*. It would appear. Not with expensive and dangerous heel injections or irreversible surgery! Body movement changes worked for me. Especially for a short-lived third attack of heel pain during a tough bike ride. I thought, *Oh! No! Not that!* I dropped my heels. Released an associated calf muscle with my thumb. Pain gone in moments!

Consider each of the dozens of recommended treatments available for so-called plantar fasciitis, on the FitOldDog Interactive Treatment Map (link). You will note that each treatment has the potential to induce major or minor modifications to one's movements. Other than that, they have little in common!

If something doesn't make sense to you, there's something you don't know!

A word to the wise.

If you experience acute morning heel pain!

Consider changing the way you think and move!

This work led me to greater interest in proprioception. A subject around which there is much debate! As Caroline Joy, an expert in body physiology, says,

Proprioception refers to the body's conscious awareness of itself ...

The proprioceptive system is responsible for maintaining reflexive control of muscle tone and posture.

As you read this, your trunk is unconsciously adjusting as your eyes shift and your head turns to read the words... your muscles perform a delicate dance of contraction and relaxation and 'restful waiting', always prepared to jump into action, without conscious deliberation or direction.

For a demonstration of Caroline Joys' points, watch the video, Wiggle Your Finger (link).

The way you move is the product of a range of reflexes. These important controls adapt to your movement choices throughout life. When you change the way you move, you are training your proprioceptive systems. Consciously or unconsciously. Changing the way you move, even subtly, can have a major impact on your movement health.

The goal of this book is to bring your movements into the light of consciousness.

This will help you to make changes in the right direction.

There's an art and a science to changing the way you think and move!

CHAPTER THREE:

THE THIRD STEP

SOLVING

In times of stringency, scientists adapt, and scientific game playing achieves new heights of precision and worth.

– Carl J. Sinderman

Remember how my Feldenkrais Instructor, Karen, worked out the source of my knee pain in 2001. Due to guarding my right ankle ever since that bike wreck in 1963. But how to solve the problem? *How to change the way I moved?* I had no idea, at the time. This problem was challenging, to say the least!

Should I pay even more money to medical professionals, coaches, or movement experts? Or could I work it out for myself and save the money? After that running-induced knee pain problem, I was skeptical of advice from medical experts!

My mind journeyed back to the fall of 1973.

It was a cold dreary day in Edinburgh, Scotland, at the Moredun Sheep Diseases Research Institute.

Surrounded by fields of sheep. An old veterinary and agricultural research facility, that carried out investigations into disease problems of sheep, cattle and goats. It was being swallowed up by the expanding city of Edinburgh and has since moved further out of town.

Everything changes with age, even institutions.

Working in these austere brick buildings for almost three years. Training to become a pathologist and researcher. I'd found my element, but was yet to master the skills needed to survive in the scientific research maelstrom. It's not the science that's the real challenge, though that's not easy. It's the people!

Humans are capricious creatures. Even supposedly logical scientists!

Hired to run the Neuropathology Diagnostic Service, I was immediately attracted to research. Not an idea I had ever entertained before! I'd just written my second scientific article, on polioencephalomalacia. A disease of the nervous system of ruminants, including sheep and cattle.

Polio = gray; Encephalon = the brain; Malacia = softening.

This work was for my doctoral degree at the University of Edinburgh. To survive in scientific research, PhD after your name can be helpful. It doesn't prove that you can think. It just convinces other people that you probably can!

Sheep affected with polioencepholomalacia fall around, tumble over, and die in seizures. They suffer a great deal in the process. These symptoms are due to gradual softening of the gray matter in their brains. Yes! Sheep have gray matter. Lots of it! We have a tendency to underestimate the intelligence of non-human animals. Especially sheep, I'm afraid! Sheep are wonderful creatures and great mothers. Based on the structure of their brains, I suspect that they enjoy fascinating dreams. How else could they stand in the heather of the Scottish hillsides, year after year. Happily chewing the cud and raising lambs? Furthermore, they can provide us with both food and clothing. Permitting humans to survive in otherwise uninhabitable regions of the planet.

The underlying mechanism, or cause, of polioencephalomalacia is a problem with vitamin B1, thiamine. This vitamin is important for our (human and sheep) bodies to turn food into energy. The brain needs lots of energy, consuming about 25% of all the energy our bodies produce. Beri-beri is the nervous dysfunction associated with vitamin B1 deficiency in humans. We are more like sheep than most people imagine.

My most recent article was rather bulky, because I'd employed a range of diverse disciplines, from the study of blood (Hematology) to brain Biochemistry.

I couldn't submit the paper to a journal for publication without the Department Heads' signature. That being Dr. Barlow. The 50 pages of text were typed on my Corona portable typewriter. The printed photos glued onto the pages. No computers in those days, not for word processing, anyway. Photographs were created using the wet chemistry methods of the day.

Digital photography was only a glint in the eye of Steven Sasson, at Eastman Kodak, back then. Black and white photography was one of my passions as a teenager. Financed with money earned on a local farm (farmhand) and in a hotel (handyman). So mastering the Pathology Department darkroom equipment was no problem. Everything you learn comes in handy one day.

Dr. Barlow accepted my precious bundle, saying, "Good work, Kevin! I'll get it back to you in about a week", which he did! Covered in red scrawl. "Not bad! Not bad at all. For your second publication! But it's too long. Much too long! I've made some suggestions."

The process was repeated, about three weeks later. To my dismay, more red scrawl: "Still too long! Kevin. Much too long!"

On the third attempt: No red scrawl, but, "Still too long! You're going to have to shorten it, or break it into two papers! I don't know how you're going to do it, but it's still much too long to publish. Sorry!"

You have to appreciate my dilemma, to understand my feelings at the time.

Publications are the currency of science. Talk is cheap, but you walk the walk with publications. Difficult to create. Based on valid data from well-designed and relevant experiments. Containing a detailed interpretation of the findings. Demonstrating a clear contribution to human knowledge. Then there's the peer review and journal editorial process. If you're challenging an established authority, this process can take years.

Believe me, I've been there!

My 'wonderful creation,' on mushy brains in sheep. Now much-improved thanks to Dr. Barlow's input, would not work as two papers. I knew it. I had removed everything I could. I liked it as it was. It was one, long, interesting and informative story!

What was I to do?

Take your mind back to the word processing technologies of the 1970s.

Sensory Input Can Be Deceiving.

Survival mechanisms kick in. I don't like Dr. Barlow's two papers advice.

A lightbulb went on. I have no idea where the idea came from, but I can guess. A book or a movie! I re-typed the whole manuscript on airmail paper. This paper is designed to reduce shipping costs. It weighs about one third that of ordinary white vellum. I also reprinted the figures on the lightest of photographic paper.

I look back on those days, from the vantage point of the more advanced technologies of today. We had a much closer relationship with each photograph. Is this worse? No! It's different. At least I didn't have to make etchings for my publications! The Victorians would have said I had it easy!

I also think that we may have had a somewhat better relationship with our bodies. In the absence of constant sensory input, from ear buds and the like.

Back to 1973:

I weighed my much lighter paper in my hand, thinking, *Will this work? Will Dr. Barlow notice? Is it honest? Is it science?*

Dr. Barlow accepted the floppy document, and didn't notice anything was amiss. Two days later he called me into his office with a smile and handed it back, unmarked. "Great work, Kevin. I enjoyed reading the shortened version. That's much better. You can submit it for publication!"

The journal accepted and published my lengthy article with little or no change. A rare event, indeed! Of course, it was submitted to the journal on regular paper!

Dr. Barlow's brain had employed the weight of the bundle of paper as a measure of the manuscript's length. This was subconscious, as he was unaware of my subterfuge. Once it had 'gone to press,' I told Dick (no longer Dr. Barlow) what I'd done, over a beer. No! I waited until the second beer. We were at our local pub, The Robin's Nest, on a Friday night after work. Celebrating the paper's acceptance by a good journal.

Dick revealed a flash of anger, as he learned what how I'd tricked him by fooling his senses.

Then, he laughed out loud and bought me another pint to toast a successful subterfuge. After all, I had provided him with another scientific publication for the department!

What had I learned from this adventure? Even experts are at the mercy of their subconscious. Including the medical professionals who saved my life from aortic disease, while advising against Ironman - was it their fear?

In that hotel room in 2010, in Barcelona, I'm clearly responsible for solving my athlete with aortic stent problem! To race or not to race, that is the question!

"It won't be solved with airmail paper," I say to myself, with a smile!

Having considered all the advice, I had to decide for myself what to do. It turns out that other athletes with stents face a similar challenge: Lack of guidance! If you are concerned, I recommend the Athletes Heart Blog, by Dr. Larry Creswell (link).

Back To Karens' Remarkable Observation.

As I left Karen, I realized that it was time to start my studies of body movement in earnest. How does a scientist do that? Reading books and articles, talking to the experts and analyzing the problem.

Running with the Whole Body: A 30-Day Program To Running Faster With Less Effort by Jack Heggie, extended my knowledge of the Feldenkrais Method. This included completing his exercises, while continuing to work with Karen.

This was followed by other books on body movement.

The Feldenkrais Teaching By Handling Method, by Yochanan Rywerant.

A Guide to Better Movement: The Science and Practice of Moving With More Skill And Less Pain by Todd R. Hargrove (the section on pain is excellent).

Anatomy Trains: Myofascial Meridians for Manual and Movement Therapists by Thomas W. Myers.

Then Continuum and Pilates were included, by excellent teachers. Rebecca Amis Lawson and Tara House, respectively. Instructive videos on YouTube provided more valuable guidance on optimal movement. Added to this were videos, made by fellow athletes of yours truly, swimming, biking and running.

It was time to do some field work. **Observing** how other people move. How they sit, stand, walk, and run. Including the movements of elite athletes. I was generally amazed and horrified by the way most people move. Especially older people. They seem bent on being bent! If they read Jack Heggie's' book, *Running With The Whole Body*, and did the exercises, they would gain so much. The majority of people seemed unaware of how they were moving around. As was I until I met Karen and The Feldenkrais Method.

By the way, fixing that knee wasn't the only expense I incurred, due to the motorcycle wreck!

Shoes of Two Different Sizes?

Most of my adult life I'd noticed that if my left foot was comfy, my right shoe was too big. If the right foot was happy, the left shoe was too tight. A thicker sock in the right shoe helped, but it felt unbalanced! Running was another matter. You need comfy, healthy, happy feet to run. Free to move in the shoe, to engage your arch machinery and avoid blisters or other aches and pains.

The solution?

Buy running shoes of two different sizes. A pair of 10s and a pair of 11s. I'd keep the 10 right and the 11 left, throwing or giving away the remaining odd pair. (Never did meet anyone needing a size 10 left and a size 11 right.)

That made 2 x $120 = $240 for a pair of running shoes!

With this solution, I was running well, picking up the pace. Cycling was also getting stronger, and it was time to buy a real triathlon bike, a custom-fit bike. I encountered Victor Jimenez of BicycleLab during a ride. He agreed to build me a bike that fit. Like shoes, your bike needs to fit, and this bike fit like a glove. Then Victor said, "Kevin, you have this great bike. Why don't you get custom bike shoes, for greater comfort and more effective interaction with the bike?"

Victor immersed my feet in a gel-like compound that set to leave a perfect impression of each foot. He sent these 'foot casts' to the shoe manufacturer. They reported that I have feet of odd sizes: 11 left, 10 right! It will cost more for the shoes. I had a good job, so we go ahead. But it got me to thinking. In fact, it got me to finally **observing** my feet. Then **questioning** the 'obvious fact' that I had genetically odd-sized feet. So could do nothing about it!

I finally noticed that my right foot with its new, more flexible ankle was all scrunched up. As part of the post-motorbike wreck, self-protection plan. Guarding! I'd been holding the little toes on my right foot in a tight bunch, for all those years. It was time to see my body movement, Continuum and dance teacher, Rebecca Amis Lawson. We had some **solving** to do.

Rebecca took one look at my right foot and said, "Kevin, you need Yoga Toes. To spread those toes and activate your arches!" Rebecca's instruction is demonstrated, in a video (link).

Within a few months, my feet were the same size. Eleven left! Eleven right!

Would you believe it? This effect is clearly demonstrated in a short video (link). Never had to buy two pairs of odd size shoes again. Running became more **affordable.**

My toes changed the way they moved!

LESSON: Never underestimate the power of guarding to screw up your life. Or that of the OQS Method to track it down and fix it! OQS helped return me to Ironman, with an AAA stent graft.

PART TWO

APPLYING THE OQS METHOD

Sitting, Standing, Walking/Running

CHAPTER FOUR

STEP FOUR

SITTING

The fall of dropping water wears away the Stone.
– Lucretius

Repetition of certain movements, consciously or unconsciously, over a life-time may have untoward consequences. They can lead to problems later in life. So beware your movement habits. One of mine ended in surgery.

A daily morning cup of tea!

About one year ago a small bump appeared near the first joint of my right index finger. On the 'thumb-ward side' of the joint. The bump was firm to the touch. A dermatologist agreed that it felt like a mass. We both suspected a giant-cell tumor, a common occurrence in this site. A hand surgeon then agreed with this diagnosis.

No choice! Finger surgery!

The surgeon kindly allowed me to watch the operation, due to my medical training. It was fascinating to see someone cutting on me while it looked as though it was someone else's finger. The magic of local anesthetic! The surgeon said, "Take a look at this, Kevin. It's a joint cyst, after all. I'll repair it, and we're done."

Time for OQS! Why had that particular part of my joint bulged?

After my hand had recovered from the surgery, I noticed a relevant issue. I was drinking my usual morning cup of tea in my favorite cup. I like a certain kind of cup handle that feels right. Residual tenderness from the surgery brought the cause to my attention. There it was! The handle of my favorite cup was resting on the surgery site. Tea cup handles had been pressing on the same region of my finger joint almost every day for over 50 years. Thousands of times! I'd worn out the joint capsule by drinking my tea in the same manner every morning.

How did I prevent re-occurrence?

By giving up my morning cuppa?

No way!

I changed the way I moved my hands around the cup.

Like drinking tea, sitting is a repetitive movement behavior!

I don't like sitting on chairs. They can put pressure on our hamstrings and even compress delicate tissues at the back of our knees. They also promote a tendency to

slump or round our backs, leading to poor posture. I always try to sit cross-legged on chairs, though it's not always possible.

There's an art to sitting. See it as another opportunity to work on your posture. To correct self-induced misalignments. I suspect that the human subjects used by designers of airplane seats have terrible posture. Head pushed forward. Body slumped. Take a look at one of those seats sometime. Posture is also incorporated into car seat design. The best one ever was the VW Rabbit Diesel. It provided firm support for the lower back, with an appropriately placed headrest.

Poor posture can drag your body earthwards. Your posture will improve if you sit up straight. Shoulders back! Your weight on your sit bones (ischial tuberosities). Face the world erect and solid in your body with good posture. This can have beneficial effects on the way you move.

There are other dangers associated with sitting for a life-time!

A major self-induced misalignment fixed by the OQS Method.

The way you start the sitting process will set up the way you sit.

Several years ago I noticed that my hips were tight on the left but not on the right. I was sitting on a bench in the gym. Facing a mirror. Right ankle resting on left knee. It felt familiar! Comfortable! OQS kicked in! *How would it feel the other way around?* Left ankle resting on right knee?

It was almost impossible to raise my left ankle onto my right knee. I had to use my hands to put it in place. My hips on that side were so tight. Then I thought, *Does this apply to the way I sit cross-legged, too?* It did! It was almost impossible to sit with my legs crossed 'the other way around.' Work to do!

Fifty years of sitting one way around had misaligned the soft tissues of my pelvis and upper legs. The effect even extended into my back and shoulders. Such self-induced misalignments accumulate over a life-time. They come home to roost eventually, leading to restricted movement. Even strains and injuries. Like a car with misaligned front wheels, leading to wear and tear on the tires and unstable road handling.

Several years of modified sitting later, either way feels normal. That left knee is still a little high. I work to coax it down, sometimes placing a weight on my left knee. Using gravity to gently lengthen those tight hip muscles.

None of us are completely symmetric. In fact, our asymmetries play a role in our attractiveness to other people. The OQS Method is designed to help you fix unhealthy asymmetries or misalignments, to prepare for aging and keep you moving.

By changing the way you move!

Transition from Sitting to Standing.

Moving from sitting to standing can be challenging, especially for older people, and from a recliner. The trick is to use gravity to your advantage. A book or other heavy object can leverage this advantage. Bring your center of gravity forward, onto your feet, by extending your arms. You then use your powerful thigh (quads) and butt (gluts) muscles to bring you to standing. With arms outstretched, you shift your center of gravity forward, away from your butt, towards your feet.

I demonstrated this method to Geneva, 89, at the mall. She was delighted, as you can see in the video, *That's So Easy* (link). Geneva later confided that she found this method really helpful when getting out of bed in the morning. I loved the smile on her face, when she found this new sense of freedom. No longer needing assistance to stand!

There are many other ways to stand up from sitting. For instance, if you have a painful lower back. Use your arms to aid your assent, as shown in the video, *How To Gete Out Of A Chair* (link).

It is well worth practicing this maneuver, before you need it in an emergency.

It's simple, really!

Just change the way you think and move!

CHAPTER FIVE

STEP FIVE

STANDING

Adapt what is useful, reject what is useless, and add what is specifically your own.

– Bruce Lee

An important skill, worth adding to your life, is the ability to calm your mind. You let go, and relax. Relaxing your mind will relax your body and improve the fluidity of your movements. It's not easy to do all the time. If you're angry for instance. Tension has a tendency to spread, to affect your whole body. Sometimes with devastating effects.

February, 1969, 3:00 am.

The phone is ringing, AGAIN! I've been working non-stop for three days and nights. Driving from farm to farm all over a 25-mile radius from our veterinary practice office. I'm all in. Not happy! Tension is building! I'm wondering if I'm cut out to be a veterinarian in clinical practice, even though most clients seem to appreciate my work. Where did that thought come from? The unhappiness was slowly growing. Unawares! I'd been in this line of work for three years. Three different jobs. This one is perfect; on duty only one night in six and one weekend in six. I still don't enjoy the work as much I thought I would. But this has been a long weekend, and the phone is ringing . . . at 3:00 in the morning.

I get out of bed, go downstairs, and stand next to the phone in the hall. With trepidation, I answer the call, thinking, *I hope it's not a difficult calving, 20 miles away. I'm exhausted!*

An elderly man's voice says, "Is that the vet?" I grunt my sleepy reply, and he says, "It's about my cat." I have no desire to leave the house again, especially on a cold night. But my job is to assist animals (and their owners!). I start the usual line of questioning about symptoms. Then I ask the question that ruined the next few days of my life:

"How long has this been going on?"

"About a week."

"And you call me at three in the morning?" I almost scream.

I was immediately angry. There was no urgency. It could wait until morning. He reacted with "Well! It's your job, and you're on duty, aren't you?" I explained that we are a small practice. There are no eight hour shifts. After-hours calls are for emergencies.

Some people are inconsiderate. At that age, my psyche was ill-equipped to cope. I reassured the man that it could wait until morning surgery. He was appeased and agreed to be there in the morning. I did manage to apologize for my frustration and calm my voice, but not my anger.

Then I felt it! Between my shoulder blades. A massive muscle spasm that confined me to my bed, unable to move, for three days. And I was just standing there. Talking! It would appear that just standing can be perilous. If you don't have your mind under control.

What was the real message my body was sending me, you might wonder? While lying in bed, unable to move, I realized that I was not in my element. I needed to seek other work, which I did. Six months later I entered a career in science, as a researcher, and never looked back. My temperament is better suited to solving scientific problems, with studies that span years. Veterinary practice deals with issues that generally take minutes to address. It also requires great people skills, while diplomacy has never been my strength.

This wasn't about a sick cat, it was about a vets' life out of whack!

When your body speaks, ask this question, *Is it a strained muscle, or is my body trying to tell me something important about my life!*

By the way, standing waiting is the perfect opportunity to work on calming your mind, improving your posture or ability to balance. As we age there is a tendency for our sense of balance to become impaired. A bad fall can finish us off! Next time you are stuck in line, pass the time by improving your sense of balance, as follows:

> *The goal of this simple exercise is to balance on one foot with the other foot barely leaving the ground. Shifting the load, gently. Unweight one foot. Feel your body tense in an attempt to maintain balance. Then relax to let your body settle its weight into balancing on one foot. Grounded. Balancing should come largely from movement around your ankles. If you lock the ankle, the balancing has to be done at the knees and hips. A less gainly task. For safety, keep the unloaded foot close to the ground.*

I do this sort of thing all the time. Standing while waiting can become your body-awareness laboratory. Use this time for stretching or some simple Feldenkrais exercises.

To change the way you move!

Transition from Standing to Walking/Running.

This is a complex topic. How this occurs will depend, to a large extent, on your walking or running skills. I recommend a combination of Danny Dryer's *Chi Running* and Jack Heggie's *Running With The Whole Body*. Falling forward from your ankles, using gravity to pull you along. Employing spinal elasticity for leg recovery, the energy to do this coming from shoulder and hip counter-rotation. In fact, spinal rigidity, with a lack of shoulder and hip rotation, appears to be one of the commonest causes of inefficient movement in adults, based on personal observations of people, as they moved around.

How you start moving will determine the way you continue to move. Be it walking or running. Watch how kids move for the best guidance. When it comes to adults, some lift their knees up and forward, using their hip flexors. Then the weight of the outstretched leg pulls their body forward. Some sway from side to side. Others shuffle along, scuffing the ground. There seem to be endless permutations of inefficient walking/running.

A short video of you moving can teach you more than all my words.

As you head off into your walk or run, think *dance*, more than *walk*. You might skip a few steps to get that lively feeling.

You can change the way you think and move!

CHAPTER SIX

STEP SIX

WALKING/RUNNING

Cats know the proper way of running for cats. Dogs and horses know the proper way of running for them, just as every human body knows the proper way of running and walking for humans. But many life conditions, ranging from poor habits, stress, injuries and impairments, a poor self-image and lack of focus, can obscure this 'forgotten knowledge.'
– Jack Heggie

December 2016.

My friend says, "I knew it was you. It's the way you walk. Why don't you walk normally. Like other people? You swing your shoulders, from side to side. I guess you do that to help your balance!" It's a statement, not a question. I don't comment as the time isn't ripe. Even though we've been meeting for lunch every couple of months for over 30 years. You have to wait until people are ready to change.

A few months later, he complains of pain in his thigh.

I say, "Where does it hurt?"

"Here," he replies, pointing at the region of a major hip flexor, the psoas muscle. "It hurts when I lift my leg." Hip flexors lift your leg!

I inform him that he's strained his major hip flexor. Explaining briefly what I've learned from Jack Heggie's book. How you can spare your hip flexors by engaging the natural spring of your spine. It turned out, based on an MRI scan, that he had also strained his *adductor longus* muscle. If you can afford such things, this is a good way to go. It could influence optimization of rehabilitation. I hasten to add that I did not suspect the *adductor longus* strain.

"Could you show me how you move?" he asks, much to my surprise! I had to wait a long time before my friend would ask for input on his movement skills. People have to be ready to change. I started to demonstrate spinal twisting, with counter-rotation of shoulders and hips, but he soon lost patience, saying, "I think I'll go to a physical therapist." Great idea if you have bottomless pockets! But what if you don't. That's one reason I wrote this book. For those who can't afford all the advantages of modern medicine!

Are you ready to change the way you move?

Tension Spreads!

One approach to learning body-awareness techniques **affordably** is to join a class. You can attend such group training for a very small fee. I recall one Feldenkrais class in which the instructor had a group of about 12 of us walking randomly around the room. Not bumping into one another. She said, "Listen to your body, and how it's moving." After a few minutes, "Now, tense your right hand."

We all noticed how our walk became stilted. Losing its fluidity, as the tension spread from our right hand throughout our bodies. We even had increased difficulty avoiding collisions.

What did we learn? Everything is connected. If you have a strained muscle, it will tend to tense up.

As a massage therapist said to me, years ago,

"Underneath tightness lies weakness!"

This is why you need both passive and active recovery. First you rest to start the repair process. When the muscle is ready, you can begin a strengthening routine.

Muscle tension can spread to adjacent, and even remote, muscle groups. I recently strained my left hip flexors. Including the *iliacus* muscle and to a lesser degree the *psoas* and *glut minimus*. Upon walking, these pesky muscles would spasm. This tension would then spread down my leg.

How to fix it?

OQS!

- **Observing**: The tension would spread if I didn't stop walking. This happened in sequence, gluts (butt muscles), hip rotators (deep hip muscles), hamstrings and finally calves. Then my left leg would lock up. I climbed on my trainer bike. To see how things responded to a light spin. I thought, "Maybe I can use active recovery to speed up repair." After five minutes at a low load, the left leg locked up. On stopping, I couldn't lift my leg. The problem was clearly centered in the muscles that lift my leg. My hip flexors!

- **Questioning:** What could be accounting for this issue? Is it a problem with my AAA stent graft. Resulting in diminished blood flow? This is dangerous! However: (1) Foot pulse is normal. (2) Nail bed refill is normal, as can be seen by simply compressing a toenail and letting go. (3) There is no swelling or discoloration. I dismissed this idea! Any doubt and I'll report to the local vascular surgery department. As 'Dirty Harry' said, "A man has to know his limitations."

- Is it a muscle spasm due to a strain or infection? If so, which muscle? As I rested the leg the tension receded from calf to hamstrings to hip rotators and finally hip flexors. Apparently, a strain of the *iliacus* and to a lesser degree the *psoas* and *glut minimus*. If I have any doubt about my diagnosis, I will report to a physical therapist that I trust.

- Can I get these muscles to let go. By applying pressure to the body (center) of each one, with my thumb? Almost immediate relief throughout my left leg. Especially with the *iliacus* and *glut minimus*. Less for the *psoas*. How about that for everything being connected!

- **Solving**: Passive recovery followed by cautious transition to active recovery.

  o Passive recovery - Rest combined with gentle thumb release and stretching several times a day.

  o Active recovery - Limited walks up to a distance that requires only one or two thumb-release sessions. Gentle spins on the bike, at low wattage, to get the blood flowing to those unhappy hip flexors.

    o   Gradual increase in exercise. Meaning never increase load, in terms of effort level or duration, by more than 10% per week. Known as the 10% rule!

It took a while to fix. Two months later, I'm up to 30-minute spins on the bike, and two-mile walks with short runs, and no release work. If all goes well, I'll be back running in a month. That is how OQS works.

Where did those tight hip flexors come from? I broke the 10% rule (link), while doing hill-climb work on a treadmill? Seemed unlikely! Eventually, it turned out that there was an underlying problem with my stent graft, restricting blood flow to my left leg. This became progressively worse, preventing me from running, comfortably. Wisely, I followed up on this contributing issue, had it repaired, and all was well again. I was training for an upcoming race, but had to pull out! Bummer! You have to go with the flow and fix things as you go along. It's all part of being an older athlete, which has it's share of excitement and disappointments.

I'm going to leave you to explore how you walk. I'll make no attempt to address your running skills, except for one important topic!

Heel Striking.

There are many runners with knees so damaged they can no longer run. Bone on bone! They all started running in their teens. They talk about how fast they were, as they hobble around today. Why? Heel striking! Landing on your heels. Even with padded shoes, running can damage cartilage in your ankles, knees and hips.

I know! I've been there when it comes to running-induced knee damage. I woke up just in time, after enjoying three knee surgeries, one as a result of a skiing accident in my 40s and the other two due to running in my 50s. Heel striking, and I had no idea.

Midlife clueless running. I was an expert!

I wised up and stopped in order to OQS the problem. This was difficult, as running is somewhat addictive. You feel so good after a long run and the costs are minimal. You can carry running gear all over the world in your hand luggage, to explore all sorts of interesting places unavailable to walkers due to time constraints.

Observing—Something is wrong with how I run. Time for the sandpit test. Simply walk or run across the sand and observe the impressions left by your running shoes. If you're heel striking, there will be a divot at the back of the impression. There it was! Heel strike!

Questioning—How can I change the way I move to prevent further damage? How do other people run without inducing damage?

Solving—I researched running styles and the causes of heel striking. I also watched hours of videos of expert runners.

Fortunately, I found Danny Dreyer of Chi Running. Chi Running seems to have nothing to do with Chi (Physical Life Force), which I studied during two years of Kung Fu in my 40s. It's real, believe you me, but it's got nothing to do with Danny Dreyer's running technique.

Danny developed an approach to walking and running that eliminates heel strike. It engages the power of gravity as you run, landing mid-foot, not on the heel. You learn to fall forward, making first contact with the ground mid-foot. You land slightly in front of your center of gravity. With a sense of falling and catching yourself, just in time. Much like kids walk and run, Danny pointed out. I combined six months of Chi Running training with the instructions of Jack Heggie in his book. *Running With The Whole Body*. This training causes you to land 'outside-midfoot.' Then to roll in towards the ball of the foot in a controlled and gentle manner (link). The goal is a soft landing using soft feet! Lowering your heel to the ground gently. Not heel striking. This provides a brief rest for your arch machinery, before the next stride.

You have to see and feel it to understand it. Watch Dennis Kimetto winning the Berlin Marathon in 2014 on YouTube. Or Loretta walking (link). Try it! Then have a friend make a video to see what you're actually doing as you walk. You may be in for a surprise.

With a lot of thought, work and observation, I changed my running style to low-impact, whole body!

The proof of the pudding is in the eating.

It turned out to be a great pudding!

I qualified for the Boston Marathon. Two years after my third and last knee surgery. Thanks to a new running style. I haven't had a heel strike-induced knee problem ever since!

I managed to change the way I moved!

Yes!!!!

Build a Growing Inventory of Body Movement Skills.

There is always more to learn as aging brings on the next challenge.

For instance, my recent chest surgery required intensive, self-directed rehabilitation for swimming. At first, *I had to change the way I moved* in the pool to avoid yanking on the incision sites. Throwing my arm more to the outside, during the recovery stroke. Rather than engaging my triceps to lift my elbows. I slowly returned to my normal stroke. Two months later everything is back in line. Swim was back. Did I pay big bucks for professional physical therapy? No! But I did apply lessons I'd learned from them, and from other sources, over the years.

Aging is not so bad so far, but it's early days in my mid-70s. I would say that my life is better in spite of it all. In fact, even an aortic aneurysm improved my life (link), believe it or not!

Aging generates interesting experiences and, thus, stories.

I noticed a tee-shirt the other day that read, "Bad decisions make good stories." Made me smile! "That can be true." I thought. "But some of our good decisions also make fascinating tales." We are a story-telling species. It's one way we gain wisdom and insights. Stories also provide inspiration. If you think you are too old to change, read *The Brain That Changes Itself,* by Norman Doidge. I came away from reading that book, and its stories, determined to keep my mind open to new ideas until the day I die.

You can change the way you think, and the way you move!

You have to believe that you can!

And do the work! It's fun!

CONCLUSION

You create your own life,

by how you see the world,

and your place in it.

– Ken Robinson and Lou Aronica

1970 in a Dusty Barn in England on a Cool Summer's Evening.

A routine visit to a remote farm in Somerset, England. To deal with a bloated sheep for a young farmer who was approximately my own age (late 20s). He was a nice chap. During the brief examination he asked me about the mechanisms of bloat. This condition causes methane gas to accumulate in the animal's rumen, a large part of the stomach. An entire ecosystem of bacteria and protozoa populate the rumen. Working together, they digest the grass. The bacteria digest the grass. The protozoa, single-celled animals, eat the bacteria. Sheep or cattle digest the protozoa.

Proto = First. Zoa = Animal.

This raises a philosophical question. "Are ruminants vegetarian if they live on protozoa?"

I digress!

Methane gas is flammable. These animals are constantly burping methane out of their mouths. This is called the eructation reflex. *Contrary to popular belief, it's not farting; it's eructation. More like burping.* I told the young farmer that the methane can be trapped as foam, due to the consumption of too much rich pasture. It became clear that I would have to use a trocar and cannula to save this sheep. Swelling of the abdomen interferes with breathing.

The astute young farmer then asked me if I'd ever ignited the gas as it escaped through the cannula. I said that I had not but would be only too willing to do so, if he was agreeable. I considered the sheep to be at no risk from what I expected to be a small blue flame.

Boys will be boys!

He clearly had this planned, much to my amusement. Reaching into his pocket, he extracted a lighter! I inserted the trocar and cannula. Once it was in place, I proceeded to remove the trocar from the hollow cannula, to release the gas.

With a grin, he had his lighter at the ready.

WOOOOOSSSHHH!

A bluish-yellow flame about eight feet long roared out of the sheep. It made us both jump, setting light to straw bales piled high behind us. With some difficulty we extinguished the blaze. Then rolled around laughing ourselves silly. The sheep was fine by the way! The story about the "young vitenry and a flaming yaw" was worth a pint or two down the local pub that night, and for years to come, I'm sure.

That flame-throwing sheep sure made us move!

Isn't this what life is about? Adventures and stories?

Let the stories continue into your golden years.

By changing the way you think and move, so you can adapt to aging with enjoyment!

EPILOGUE

Of Heroes and Inspiration

Frits With An S.

As I mentioned previously, I met Frits on our bikes, at the 2010 Lake Placid Ironman. We encountered each other again the following year in Lake Placid and at the World's Half Ironman Championships in Las Vegas in 2013. Recently, to my delight, Frits agreed to act as my coach, using his "secrete sauce," for my next Ironman race. Frits was a dedicated student and coach of Ironman triathlons. He studied every aspect. He did admit that he hated swimming, but he did it anyway. As a life-long swimmer, I find this interesting. I know several other triathletes with this problem. I suspect it's related to learning to trust the water. That's my guess, anyway!

Frits passed away recently, leaving me with fond memories and lots of sadness. Deb and I still have a good friend, Frits's wife, Machteld, who we visited in the Netherlands, recently. This will allowed us to say goodbye to Frits properly . . . over a meal, and a toast in Frits's honor, of course!

Bob Scott.

"Bob Scott had chest pain during a bike ride a decade ago and did what any triathlete would do. He rode his bike to his doctor's office. After an examination, his suspicions of cardiac disease confirmed, the doctor wanted Scott to head to the hospital for a cardiac cath. Scott agreed and started to put his helmet back on to ride his bike to the hospital. The doctor would have none of it and Scott was transported in the usual fashion. After a stent placement and recovery, he went on to set the Kona age group records for the next age group (75-79)"—John Post

At age 81, Bob came by me on the run in the Maryland Half Ironman. I was in my late 60s and pretty fit. He beat me again when he was 82 and again at 84. He said a friendly, "Hi, Kevin," as he cruised by each time. Bob has mastered the art of aging! He loves doing what he does! He's in his element!

Sure inspires me to keep going!

Pauline Carol Watson.

I started my blog, Athlete With Stent, in 2010. About six months later, I heard from my first athlete with aortic disease, Pauline. There aren't too many us!

I received Pauline's introductory comment on a blog post. Having a 4.8 cm. diameter AAA, Pauline said she found my blog encouraging. Pauline is a talented and avid runner as is her supportive husband, Bob. In 2013, they kindly drove from Toronto to Cleveland to treat me to dinner a couple of days before my second aortic surgery. We raced together in 2015, at the Eagleman Half Ironman in Cambridge, Maryland. It was my pleasure to be trounced by Pauline, who I admire a great deal.

How I Feel when I compete in an Ironman Race.

Each time I train for and undertake one of these grueling races, the feelings are the same. I wouldn't miss it for the world. Aortic disease or no aortic disease. I'll just keep going for as long as it is safe to do so, and I enjoy the process.

I feel the **excitement** of the challenge, the **enjoyment** of a solid workout, the **sense of being alive,** while running in a thunderstorm in a foot of water, the **dismay** of surgery, the **exhaustion** of a category one bike climb leading to a **sense of awe** at the cyclists in the Tour de France that can only come from completing such a climb, the **fear** of failure or crashing on a long descent, the **disappointment** of a poor performance, the **nausea of bonking**, the **anxiety** about being twice the age of almost everyone else in Ironman training camp including the coach, the **anger of hypoglycemia** (low blood sugar), the **pride** of a better swim time in the pool, the **wonder** of swimming with dolphins in Hawaii permitted by a high level of fitness, the **confusion** of a problem unsolved, the **delight** in finding the answer, the **trepidation** of race-day morning on the beach, the **happiness** of hearing my family and friends supporting me from the side-lines, the

relief of reaching the finish line, the **pain** in my thighs as I struggle back to my tent, the **explosion of flavors** in my mouth from the best food in the world, the **satisfaction** of a well-earned beer handed to me by a friend, the **appreciation** for my support team and great coaches, the **gratefulness** to my son, Nigel, for introducing me to this fascinating sport, the **calm** of a good night's sleep and awakening the next day to the **anticipation** of planning my next race.

Go out there and find your element.

Create your stories to tell friends in the pub. Relate to your grandchildren. Or to delight in as fond memories of a job well done!

You may have to change the way you think and the way you move!

POST-SCRIPT

Until you value yourself,

you won't value your time.

Until you value your time,

you will not do anything with it. – M. Scott Peck

Two Of My Family's Favorite Stories, About Pride And Imagination.

They relate to avoiding unhealthy pride, while fostering your imagination. You need both humility and imagination to take on the task of *changing the way you think and move (and feel, for that matter!).*

Pride!

Pride goeth before a fall. –

Misquote from The Book of Proverbs

It's 1970 on a farm in Somerset, England.

A routine call to a cow having trouble delivering her calf. The farmer, a huge man, is standing in a field near the gate as I drive in. I was young-looking, fair-haired, not so tall, and round-faced with lots of auburn hair. But I had three years of intense veterinary experience under my belt.

I climbed out of my car and approached the hostile giant of a man. He looked down at me and said, "I see they're sending children to treat my stock. Can't someone more experienced deal with this? It's a difficult case, and she's a valuable milker. Gave over 2,000 gallons last year."

This was a familiar story! I ignored his comment and said, "Good evening, Mr. Adams. Please fetch me a bucket of hot water. Then take her head, and we'll see what's going on!"

He stalked off while I examined a stressed mother to be. She looked at me with frightened eyes as she strained to deliver her youngster. She was a lovely animal, but it was pouring with rain, soaking us both to the skin. On examining this massive cow, I found an over 100-lb calf that was alive but impossible to deliver.

I'd delivered many difficult calves with calving ropes and a little patience. It was not to be, this time. "She'll need a Caesarean," I said, "but it won't take long." This farmer cared about his cows. He didn't hesitate to spend the money on his livestock, while having serious reservations about me.

I extracted my gear from the car and sterilized the surgical instruments in a little boiler designed for the job. I then laid everything on a clean towel on a bale of straw next to the expectant mother. She was a large, good-tempered animal.

It was still pouring with rain as I started the operation! I handed the truculent farmer a large umbrella and told him to hold it over the operation site. So I could see what I was doing. It really was a deluge, but that cow couldn't wait!

He seemed to think that holding the umbrella was below his station. He complied out of pure curiosity, I'm sure. I gave the cow a tranquilizer to keep her calm and standing still. Then I applied a nerve block so that she wouldn't feel my incisions. And on I went, enjoying my work, which was satisfying in many ways.

I shaved and sterilized the incision site and made my first cut, about 15 inches long, through the skin. Remember, that calf weighed more than a hundred pounds. It was big! On making the incision, I sensed movement behind me. I turned to see the farmer, still holding up the umbrella. But he was falling like a felled tree. He missed the cow and me, but his inert body crashed onto the sterilised instruments.

Into the mud went the whole mess, farmer and all.

With some difficulty, I dragged his inert body to an adjacent tree and propped him up. He'd passed out from the sight of blood. I hurried to find his wife, a tiny woman with lively eyes and a quick wit. She told me that her husband was a big milksop, and she was not at all surprised about the mess he'd created. Within 20 minutes, we had sterilized the instruments again. With the lady of the house holding the umbrella, I delivered a healthy, heifer calf in the rain. The farmer recovered from his fall, his only injury being dented pride. Then we all had a cup of tea to celebrate the delivery in their nice, warm kitchen.

Even Mr. Adams smiled at me and laughed about our adventure.

Lesson learned: Judge people by their actions rather than their words or appearance. Clearly, my actions overcame the resistance of Mr. Adams to my apparent youth and inexperience.

Imagination

I believe that imagination is stronger than knowledge.

That myth is more potent than history.

That dreams are more powerful than facts.

That hope always triumphs over experience.

That laughter is the only cure for grief.

And I believe that love is stronger than death.

– Robert Fulghum

Negative Socks!

I enjoy chatting with my stepson Nick. Great athlete, wonderful person and deep thinker! One day, Nick and I are leaving the mall, and we pass a 19 mph speed limit sign. It always attracts my attention because of an interest in prime numbers. Nineteen is one of my favorites.

I was reminded of an excellent book on the subject: *Prime Obsession: Bernhard Riemann and the Greatest Unsolved Problem in Mathematics* by John Derbyshire. The chapters alternate: One on a part of Riemann's brief life and the next addressing the mathematics needed to understand the Riemann Hypothesis on prime number theory. The math is provided step-wise in a comprehensible manner.

I mentioned this to Nick. He's a bright kid, but he gave me a look, as if to say, "Yep! You're weird, Kevin."

Before seeing that speed limit sign, Nick and I had been having a conversation about socks. We were at the mall to buy shoes as his were now too tight. His foot size reminds me of a Giacometti statue; he is going to be tall. In the store, Nick had explained that his shoes had been too tight for a while. So I suggested that he buy some negative socks.

I received an odd look, and he said "What?"

"Well, Nick!" I replied. "If your shoes are too big, you can put on thick socks to fill up the extra space, and they'd feel better, right? They are positive socks!" He nodded in agreement. I then said, "They fill up, or take away, actual or positive space in your shoes. But if you had negative socks, they would add space. Then your tight shoes would be looser and more comfortable. Right?" He looked puzzled for a moment, and then the light went on, and it got him thinking, which was what I was trying to do in the first place.

The idea of negative socks came to me from a couple of sources, one being the negative space used for improving drawing skills. This has been used effectively in advertising. Look at the FedEx sign, and notice the large arrow, written in negative space, in their logo. The other source was my interest in "inner space" as a kid. If you can go outwards to infinity, why not inwards too? This idea used to fascinate me. I would imagine worlds within worlds within worlds.!

The Universe is an odd place. It pays to question everything even the obvious absence of negative socks. In long races, on hot days, my feet swell a bit. I sure would like to have a pair of negative socks in my pocket. In fact, I could store things in them, such as extra food and more pairs of negative socks.

APPENDIX A

ON BALANCE

Balance is a double meaning word; you need balance to stand up and not fall, but you need balance in your life areas, or else your life will become unstable.

– Mr. Myagi, *The Karate Kid*

Balanced Movement: Your movements depend, to a large extent, on your sense of balance. Your brain uses several sources of information to enable you to sit or stand safely. This information is critical when you negotiate complex movements in dangerous environments!

- The inner ear senses direction and orientation of motion.

- Somatic senses detect pressure and tension in muscles and joints. This aspect of balance is aided by a strong, flexible body. This is one reason weight-training is of value for active, healthy aging.

- Vision allows us to use fixed objects to determine our location in space. This is why it is more difficult for us to balance with our eyes closed.

- Receptors on the soles of our feet sense our relationship to the ground. Shoes, especially modern, padded trainers, have 'blind-folded' our feet. Reducing our ability to read the ground, which may impair our sense of balance.

There are many ways to improve your sense of balance. This work will allow you to reduce the risk of life-threatening falls and stumbles, as you age.

Aids to balance include a walking stick or walker. Let's put that off for as long as we can! Then we can lean on walls or furniture, a common strategy. Yoga Toes can spread your feet and activate your arches, for better balance (link). I've recently been testing a new product, VOXXLife Socks (link). These comfortable socks are designed to activate receptors on the soles of our feet. Improving balance and athletic performance. They are yielding promising results for people with balance issues, such as those suffering from multiple sclerosis (MS). I'm sure such inventions will improve with time.

That said, I recommend that you hone your balance skills. I have done so to good effect for triathlon training. For instance, the best swimmers perfect their balance in the water. This makes relaxed swimming almost effortless. You will learn to improve your balance from back-to-front and side-to-side. The *Total Immersion Swimming Program* teaches this process.

You neglect your sense of balance, at your peril, as you age!

Balanced Life: Here's another critical balance issue, when it comes to your health and aging. That between blindly accepting advice from health professionals *versus* deciding for yourself.

Valium? Yes please, doctor.

We can experience loss of balance while looking down from tall buildings. In response to severe dehydration. And increasingly as we age. Age-related vertigo can be crippling and is not to be underestimated as a health challenge. If you suffer from vertigo for no apparent reason, try the Epley Maneuver (link). It just might work for you.

I recently suffered a severe case of vertigo, accompanied by uncontrollable vomiting. This resulted from training-related dehydration. I completely lost my sense of balance and started to retch violently. Only one thing really helped in the short term. Valium administered in an ambulance. I would normally avoid such a dangerous drug like the plague. But valium worked wonders for my vertigo and led to cessation of the vomiting. This resulted in my ability to drink fluids and all was well, eventually. I learned a lot that day including the dangers of bonking out of context (link).

Valium? No thanks, doctor!

Many people, it would seem, want an external agent, doctor or pill, to fix their pain. They want them to fix things now and as conveniently as possible. For a minor headache this might work. For temporomandibular joint (TMJ) pain? It's another story.

I suffered from this painful condition about 15 years ago. Thinking it was swimmer's ear, I went to a doctor for some antibiotics. A nice young physician looked in my ear and said, "It's not your ear, Kevin; it's TMJ. Are you stressed about something, grinding your jaws at night?" He simultaneously started writing on his prescription pad.

What are you writing a prescription for?

He replied, "Valium to calm you down. A strong anti-inflammatory to protect the joint!"

I replied, "I appreciate it, but no thanks! I'll take a week's vacation and both meditate and sleep a little more. This is a warning sign that my life is out of control."

The young doctor looked puzzled. He insisted on handing me the prescriptions, which I later tore up and threw away. Within two weeks, following my own treatment plan, the TMJ pain was gone – I was body and mind aware enough to know warning signs.

Sure, the drugs would have helped me continue my stressful lifestyle. And later take me towards a heart attack.

Listen to those warning signals! Your life may depend upon it!

Doctors can be great, but they aren't always right!

Hesitate before reaching for those pills.

It may be better to change the way you think, move and live your life!

APPENDIX B

CLIFFS NOTES

APPROACH TO OQS

Insanity: doing the same thing over and over again, and expecting different results.
– Albert Einstein

I'm assuming that you are taking good care of your nutrition and enjoying adequate sleep? If you awake stiff and sore with a crick in your neck, apply OQS!

You may have to change the way you move in bed!

OQS And Health Challenges—The OQS Method grew out of my desire to continue Ironman training with aortic disease. I realized that I would have to change the way I moved. The wrong move could kill me. Literally! You may have your own health challenges to consider. If you're in doubt about how to proceed, read, *Sport Benefit Risk Analysis: Rediscovering Your Sport Safely After A Major Health Challenge* (link).

OQS And Aging—Successful aging is about adaptation to change.

OQS And Our Individual Uniqueness—We each have our own psychological, genetic, social, nutritional and injury history. When it comes to mobility as we age, one size of treatment does not fit all, thus the need to carefully observe, question and solve.

Fighting Aging Body Aches and Pains.

There is no limit to how much money you can spend on avoiding or curing body aches and pains. As a lifetime athlete, I've invested thousands. I don't regret one cent, but I had a good job at the time. We each have to decide for ourselves when it comes to the use of limited resources. I finally concluded that many of my pains, sprains and injuries were avoidable, *if only I'd changed the way I moved.*

What is best for you and your goals? You could go with the most popular, such as yoga. This is available almost everywhere in the USA. The more effective introduction to body-movement training, Feldenkrais, is almost an open secret. There are many others including Pilates, Continuum, The Alexander Technique, a range of Martial Arts, Gyrokinesis, and a growing number of

Integrated Medicine programs that include some movement training.

If you complete steps 1-5 below, and no more, you will gain enormous benefit. IF you carry out all of the exercises in *Jack Heggie's remarkable book!* After that, the sky's the limit when it comes to movement training.

Consider the process an investment rather than an expense, and you will reap the benefits. You may save a bunch on medical bills!

1. **($0.00) Make your injury map** and include any issues that may influence your long-term physical health including diet, genetic history and physical damage from accidents. An example is provided in the video, FitOldDog's Injury Map: For Active Healthy Aging (link).

2. **($0.00) Have a friend make short videos** of you sitting, getting up from sitting, standing, starting to walk, walking, and running (if you're a runner). Examine the video to see how you actually move. Keep it for future reference to gauge your progress.

3. **($0.00) Learn to work your core safely** by watching *Body Movement for Aging: The Art Of Stretching For Flexibility As You Age* (link).

4. **($0.00) Watch Feldenkrais videos on YouTube.** It also helps to keep a diary of how you feel. Learn how to observe your movements more closely.

5. **($2-5 for a second-hand copy) Even if you have no interest in running, buy a copy of Jack Heggie's book** *Running With The Whole Body* and complete the 30 lessons. Make notes in the book or a diary. It's the least expensive and most effective introduction to body-awareness that I know. It will introduce you to the Feldenkrais Method. This will start you down the road to building a body-awareness training routine. Make it a habit, and it will stick!

6. **($30) Find an inexpensive movement class** and ask the instructor if they could focus on core for one lesson. Don't overdo it; pace yourself. The aim is for you to get to know your core. It's the center of your physical power and ability.

7. **($40) Find your weakest link(s).** Book a 30-minute appointment with a massage therapist, which may be free. Ask the massage therapist to tell you which muscles are tight and what other issues need addressing. My issue was lack of freedom of movement of my

shoulder blades. Feldenkrais helped me to fix this (link) several years later.

8. **($100) Find your next weakest link(s).** Book an appointment with a physical therapist for an assessment. A physical therapist identified weak adductor muscles in my legs. I had no idea! It gave me something to focus on before trouble erupted.

9. **($24) Take one or two group Feldenkrais classes** as you can learn a lot from watching other students.

10. **($100 + $50/month) Join your local gym or YMCA** (where financial aid is available). Use the mirrors for form. Ask advice of staff. Develop your weight training program. Collect ideas from other members, selecting people who know what they are doing. NOTE: I did not say a weight-lifting program. I recommend light weights and lots of repetitions for conditioning as you age. This is a risk-free way to strengthen weak bones, muscles, connective tissue and joints. It also helps to prevent osteoporosis when combined with good posture. Tailor your workouts to your sport. For instance, I use swim cords in the gym for triathlon training.

Create your own routine, and you'll be more likely to stick to it. Incorporate walking, running, canoeing or any other exercise you enjoy!

Learn how to change the way you think and move as you go along!

APPENDIX C

STRAINS AND INJURIES

I'm not a doctor or physical therapist. I'm a veterinarian, working to help you fix strains and injuries as affordably as possible. If you are in any doubt as to your strain or injury, seek professional medical advice.

It's up to you how you handle strains and injuries. This is what I do based on 60 years of sports and countless minor, and not so minor, self-inflicted injuries.

1. **Stop,** as soon as I detect an issue. This may occur as much as several days after I did the damage. Sometimes I know I'm doing damage, and I don't know how I know. Experience and training, I guess. If there is any doubt, I stop. Never attempting to run through the pain.

2. **Observe** the damage, looking for signs of swelling, bleeding or inflammation. I also consider how the painful area feels and how it affects other areas of my body.

3. **Question** and wonder what led up to the problem. Was there any change in my workouts? Was I particularly tired before my training? I look back, trying to find anything

that might have accounted for the issue. Generally, many small events add up to create a strain or injury. For instance, in 1986, at the Snow Shoe Ski Resort in North Carolina, I damaged my left knee. I tore my medial collateral ligament and split the medial meniscus. This resulted in corrective surgery two years later. What were the events that led up to this? (1) Weak bones and joints due to mild rickets as a kid, (2) Brand-new, and thus unfamiliar, skis and boots, (3) A full-day ticket for the first day of the skiing season and I skied all day, (4) Distraction; talking to a friend as we drifted along the almost flat path back to the lodge. My skis close together, with tired legs. The left ski caught an edge, and slid off into mushy powder on the side of the trail, and immediately stuck. Because of tiredness, my left knee was straight. Bad decision! There was a sound like the breaking of a chicken neck. My skiing days were over. It was 1986, but the injury was set up many years before. During World War II. Back in 1943-1948. In Bristol, England, where most of us kids had poor nutrition during a critical growth period!

4. **Solve or attempt to solve,** by putting together the pieces of the puzzle. If I'm unable

to work out what is going on, I seek medical advice. You might be thinking, *I'd just go to see my doctor!* I then would ask you, "And which kind of doctor are you going to select?" This is a critical question. Say you have a pain in your foot! Do you go to a family doctor? Sports physician? Podiatrist ? Chiropractor? Acupuncturist? Feldenkrais Instructor? Massage Therapist? Or your local shoe store? Even socks can cause severe foot pain. Especially over-tight tube socks! The wrong decision could take you down a multi-thousand-dollar road. It did for me! An injury map could have saved me a lot of trouble and expense. Given that my knee problem was on the same leg that had been broken in the motorbike wreck many years before. This is why good record-keeping can help to solve problems. It often works in science, so maybe it will work for your strain or injury.

5. **Consider all the options** when it comes to treatment. Most people will go to the first medical professional that pops into their head. Or one they are familiar with! They generally do this without a prior analysis of their issue. We are problem-solving creatures, designed to rush in and 'fix it' to survive. As David Kord Murray

explains in his book *Borrowing Brilliance: The Six Steps to Business Innovation by Building on the Ideas of Others:*

> *You're wired for speed, not precision. Imagine your ancient ancestor. Observing the rustling of the grass approaching him on the prehistoric savannah. This was either a saber-toothed tiger or the wind blowing the tall grass. The ancestor who made a quick decision to run, was the one who survived. Passing this trait to you. The one who stayed to determine the source of the rustling grass, was more apt to be eaten by the tiger. His genes, and aptitude for problem analysis, were taken out of the gene pool, long before modern times.*

A sore foot is not a saber-toothed tiger!

If necessary stop completely, and start over. Use beginner's mind. This takes discipline but it got me to the Boston Marathon in 2009.

How about you?

What adventure do you plan to undertake?

Now that you've learned how to change the way you think and the way you move!

APPENDIX D

SUGGESTED READING

Selected movement exercises are presented on the FitOldDog YouTube Channel (link).

If you are prepared to read only one book:

Running With The Whole Body: A 30-Day Program to Running Faster with Less Effort by Jack Heggie, 1996. NOTE: It works just as well for walking!

If you would like to dig a little deeper into healthy body movement:

A Guide to Better Movement: The Science and Practice of Moving With More Skill And Less Pain by Todd R. Hargrove, 2014.

Want to dig even deeper:

The Feldenkrais Teaching By Handling Method, by Yochanan Rywerant, 1981.

Anatomy Trains: Myofascial Meridians for Manual and Movement Therapists, 3e by Thomas W. Myers, 2014.

Proprioceptive Training: A Review of Current Research by Caroline Joy Co, 2010.

Consider reading these other books for active healthy aging:

Healthy Aging: A Lifelong Guide to Your Well-Being by Andrew Weil, 2007.

You don't believe you can change the way you think? Think again!

The Brain That Changes Itself: Stories of Personal Triumph from the Frontiers of Brain Science by Norman Doidge, 2007.

More relevant reading for happy healthy active aging:

Finding Your Element: How to Discover Your Talents and Passions and Transform Your Life by Ken Robinson and Lou Aronica, 2014.

Tao Te Ching by Lao-tzu (4th c. BCE), translated by Steven Mitchell, 1994.

The Power of Now: A Guide to Spiritual Enlightenment by Eckhart Tolle, 2004.

The Three Minute Meditator: Reduce Stress. Control Fear. Diminish Anger. In Almost No Time at All. Anywhere. Anytime by David Harp, 2008.

The Road Less Traveled, Timeless Edition: A New Psychology of Love, Traditional Values and Spiritual Growth by M. Scott Peck, 2003.

Borrowing Brilliance: The Six Steps To Business Innovation By Building On The Ideas Of Others by David Kord Murray, 2010.

All Creatures Great And Small by James Herriot, 1998.

Winning The Games Scientists Play by Carl J. Sindermann, 2001. A must for young scientists!

Zen And The Art Of Motorcycle Maintenance, An Inquiry Into Values by Robert M. Pirsig, 2006.

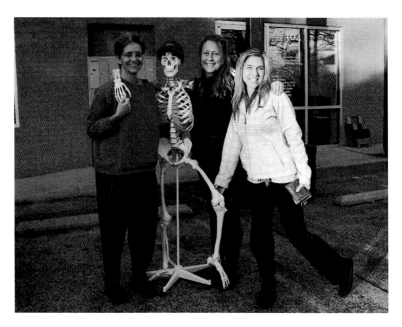

The author's key movement instructors, Left to right, Karen,
Mr. Bones, Rebecca and Tara.

ACKNOWLEDGMENTS

I gained considerable assistance with body movement and athletic training from a long list of people. My key body-awareness insights, for which I am extremely grateful, were drummed into my skull by three wonderful movement educators: Karen Dold, Rebecca Amis Lawson and Tara House.

I also wish to thank those who both encouraged and aided me with preparation of this book, along with their comments on my cover design, including Sarah, Heather, Myles, Deb and Sue.

Thank y'all so much, especially the people I forgot to mention.

kev!